Nothing to See
and Nothing to Feel

Christina Peters-Smith

authorHOUSE®

AuthorHouse™ UK Ltd.
500 Avebury Boulevard
Central Milton Keynes, MK9 2BE
www.authorhouse.co.uk
Phone: 08001974150

First published by AuthorHouse 1/19/2010

ISBN: 978-1-4490-0989-2 (sc)

This book is printed on acid-free paper.

CHAPTER 1

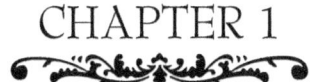

Have you ever had one of those days when you are told something that is like a bolt out of the blue and your words are "Why Me?" well - why not me - what makes me any more special or different to any other person - and it is ME today and I have to get on with it.

So this is my story - I am not going to bore you with my life before Cancer - just my life leading up to and hopefully past.

On my 51st birthday - I could not understand why I had not received an "Invitation" for a Breast Cancer Screening - as in 2001 it was quite the thing that on your 50th birthday it was advisable for all women to be screened.

At that time I was living in Bristol and contacted the Breast Cancer Clinic. I went for my mammogram only to have a letter to say that there were some "abnormalities" and could I please return.

At this time of my life I was divorced and living with my daughter and so she came to the Clinic with me. The x-rays showed that there was a "calcification" (which I will explain later) in the left breast - so they advised me to have a biopsy. Also at this time in my life my mother was alive and although I had tried to keep all this from her until it was all over - you know what us mum's are like - we just know when there is something wrong.

Anyway following the biopsy (which was not at all pleasant) having shot me in the left breast twelve times with only what I can describe as a gun similar to that of piercing your ears (but unfortunately you are not left with a pretty sparkling ear-ring at the end of it) I then had to return to be given the results.

My daughter - mum and dad came with me - it was like a little family outing. Anyway - the result of all that was - following a second screening - that I was in the clear! Oh what a relief - my mum burst into tears and obviously my dad's first reaction was - there is a problem but we will over come it together - it was not until we told him that I was in the clear that he asked us why we had been crying - men!!

I then met a very special man in my life - and I decided that I did not want to remain on my own - my daughter was getting older and would soon be flying the nest - my son had found himself a lovely young lady to settle down with (they are now married with a beautiful little girl and a two week old baby son) and so I decided to rent my house in Bristol - move to Cheltenham to be with Keith - which worked out so well that after six months I decided to sell up my home.

We had been really happy - everything just seemed to be going well apart from about two years ago - for whatever reason I just did not feel 100% - I did not feel ill but I just did not feel right.

My son was getting married in 2006 and I wanted to look and feel my best for the wedding - but whatever it was that was wrong would just not let me get on top of it - and I kept it to myself that I was just not feeling the best.

My left arm at the top kept swelling and I went back for my usual breast scan (as they were keeping a close eye on me now) as I had a history of three aunts on my dad's side with breast cancer and a cousin (who has unfortunately just died) with the same disease.

I have an amazing Breast Cancer Surgeon (Mr Bristol) who gave me a thorough examination - there was nothing to be detected on any of the mammograms - and he just informed me that due to my age the inside of my breasts were like "a bag of broken biscuits" - great!

Anyway - just to be on the safe side in February 2007 I had to go for an MRI scan - purely because they could not understand why the top of my left arm kept swelling - but that was not as simple as it sounds either.

I went in for the scan (feeling absolutely terrified) as it was a full body scan taking about 45 minutes and not being able to move at all - the most awful sensation I think I have ever experienced in my life – it felt as though I was being pounded by an air cushion underneath me - to find after about 35 minutes the door being opened and me being pulled out as quickly as possible - fire alarms going off - to be informed that the alarms were showing the scanner was on fire (I know whilst I was lying there I was praying to my mum - who had unfortunately passed away by this time - to give me a sign that she was looking after me and going to take care of me through this traumatic experience - I did not expect the sign to be that dramatic!)

After we had all sat outside for a while - the fireman and fire engines etc had all gone - we were to find out later that workman upstairs had apparently done something that had affected the alarm to the scanner - that should have been my first "Why Me"

Anyway - results came back from the MRI - absolutely clear. Nothing abnormal at all. So - we continue to get on with our lives and now Keith and I had decided that we are going to get married on the 19th July 2008 and we both realised that we had put on a little weight due to contentment - so we spend £500 and join the gym.

We go for our first assessment for me to be told that it would be advisable for me to go and see a doctor straight away, as my blood pressure was sky high. I went to the doctor the next day to be signed off work immediately for the week, to be advised that my blood pressure was so high that I could go at any time - I just had to stay at home and relax. As not only do we have a history of breast cancer in the family - my brother at the age of 40 had a massive heart-attack and has since had a quadruple by-pass and my mother who had a pneumovax injection on the Monday morning was dead by the Monday afternoon, after having suffered a major heart attack (and bless her heart, I was only talking and laughing with her on the Sunday, as they were coming up to visit us on the following Friday) - they say you should never take life for granted as you never know what will happen from one day to the next.

Anyway - I digress - I stayed at home and I was monitored by the doctors - still having high blood pressure and high cholesterol - so now on two tablets a day for that.

Feeling better - I returned to the gym and decided to have a Personal Trainer (Sally) - who carried out a full assessment on me and yes - it looked as though it was all systems go and I was going to be fit and trim for my wedding a few months away and so I paid my £100 and got my training schedule (and Sally has kept in constant contact with me during my rough times) bless her.

Guess what - no that did not happen either - because just before I was due to start my training- I did not feel at all well at work - and had been suffering very bad night sweats - but knew it could not be the change (as that was one thing I had already gone through).

Went to the doctor the next day - to be informed immediately that again my blood pressure was sky high - but that I also had a virus - so to stay at home and have complete rest. What is going on with me - it seems that from the moment we said we were going to get married everything seemed to be going wrong.

Well, the wedding was fast approaching and everything had to be sorted - so I just got on with organising that - the virus seemed to have gone and I was feeling not too bad - during which time I had decided to stop taking the tablets.

Keith and I had a double appointment to see the doctor - who asked me "why are you not taking the tablets" - to which I replied "I hate tablets and I am not going to take them" to which she replied "Chris - you have two choices, you either take the tablets and live - or you don't take the tablets and you will die" - not much of a choice then really was there - so needless to say under duress I took the tablets and with the wedding getting ever closer, I was beginning to feel quite well - not 100% but better than I had felt for a long time.

CHAPTER 2

We got married on the 19th July - had a fabulous time (although there always has to be someone to spoil the day but at this stage I am not going to bore you with those details) and we then flew off to Antigua for two weeks honeymoon (which also had a dampener put on it as the person who spoilt our wedding day was also playing on Keith's mind whilst we were away - he could not understand why this particular person had been so cruel to do what they did). But again I am not going to waste my time telling you that side of the story. It was just so awful to see Keith so disappointed and very down.

When we returned I had a letter from the Mobile Mammogram Clinic to attend for a routine mammogram on the 21st August 2008. To which I attended obviously. On Thursday 28th August I received a letter from the Breast Clinic to say that there were some abnormalities and would I go for a further appointment on Monday 1st September. I just burst into tears - Keith was in the garden watering the plants and I just sobbed and sobbed - he then realised there was something wrong and came in and cuddled me - I told him that "I knew there was something wrong" - I just felt it in myself.

I had my dad coming for the weekend - who usually arrives on the Friday and leaves on the Monday - but I asked him if he would mind going back on the Sunday as I knew I was not going to be in a good frame of mind and I did not want to upset him.

I went to the Breast Clinic on Monday 1st September - went in for mammograms at 9.30 - Keith and I were called into the Doctor who showed us the x-rays and we were told that there were three calcifications (you can have a macro calcification or an micro calcification) in the left and a lump in the right - but at that stage there did not seem to be anything sinister - they even did the breast scan whilst Keith was there. Keith went back out into the waiting room whilst they did the biopsies.

Now this is where the difference comes in between a calcification and a lump. Can I also say at this stage that for myself (or the doctor) there is nothing to see and nothing to feel on either breast and no abnormality in shape. So first reaction is that everything is fine because there is Nothing to See and Nothing to Feel! How wrong we were.

The doctor carried out the first biopsy on the right breast (which is where the lump was) and this biopsy was done by the doctor with the body scanner because the lump could be seen on the monitor. They took four shots of the right breast - bearing in mind this takes a lot of prodding and pushing and inserting needles before they shoot the gun. Yes - they got the samples that they wanted - but by this time it was now about 11.15 and they thought it was time to give my body a rest, so to go and sit in the waiting room with Keith and have a cup of tea and they would then call me in ten minutes and they would then do the left breast (poor Keith by this time was now of the belief I was all finished and we were going home).

The left breast needed to be done with the mammogram machine, because this is the one with the calcifications and they do not show up on the body scanner. Macro-calcifications are coarse calcium deposits in the breast. They look like large white dots or dashes on a mammogram. They are a natural result of breast ageing and are found in about half of women over the age of 50 and in about 1 in 10 younger women. They may be caused by calcium deposits in a cyst, or in milk ducts, as women get older. They may also be the result of previous injuries or inflammation. Calcium in the diet does not cause calcifications.

Apparently macro-calcifications are harmless and are not linked with cancer so they do not need any treatment or monitoring. Micro-calcifications are tiny calcium deposits and show as fine white specks on a mammogram. This is where the cells are being replaced more quickly than normal. Usually, micro-calcifications are not due to cancer, but in a small number of cases, a group of micro-calcifications which are in a cluster may be a sign of pre-cancerous changes in the breast, or of an early breast cancer.

The doctor took three shots at the left breast purely because of the fact that there were three calcifications which they had to try and get samples of. Again a lot of pulling and pushing and fitting you into the machine and then it is all done digitally and once they have the breast in the right place the gun is shot from the machine.

I might as well state at this point as well that I was a 38C (but obviously not now!)- so there is quite a lot there to be pulled and prodded around - plus the tissue inside the breast is quite dense and so quite difficult to penetrate.

Well, the doctor has now got the samples that she needs to send to the Lab and I am just sitting there - naked from the waist up - waiting to be told that I can get dressed and go home and that they will be in touch.

No - it was not going to be as easy and straight forward as that. The doctor came into the room and she looked upset and her words to me were "what is it about the thought of a mastectomy that you do not like" and I told her that my aunts had had one years ago and that I did not like the way that my body would look once the surgery was over. She told me that they had come on leaps and bounds now and that the reconstruction work was absolutely brilliant and the survival rates were high.

So I told her that if it was a case of removing the diseased breast and that I would be cancer free and survive - then so be it - she then hit me with the double mammy, it was apparent that there was a problem in both breasts and I would have to have a double mastectomy! - I just felt numb for a few seconds and then came back with - well I am going to take a positive approach to this and if this is what has to happen then so be it.

I went into the waiting room and got Keith - walked into the car park and of course by this time he is still thinking that everything is fine (because that is what he had last heard the doctor say). When I burst into tears and told him what she had just said (that I had cancer) he was as numb as me I think.

We came home and I had promised to call my daughter and my dad straight away but only if it was bad news - if good I would ring them in the evening. I did not come out of the Clinic until about 1.15 - by which time everyone had thought that it was obviously good news.

9

I rang my daughter - and bless her heart she just broke down and said that she was coming straight up - my dad did not reply so I left a message. Eventually he rang me and I broke the news and he broke down as well (making me feel really bad because he lives alone in Devon) but I knew that he had a lot of good friends that he could go to.

My daughter arrived not long after and we both had a very caring - sharing and tearful moment. We then decided that this was not the way forward and whatever was going to be it was going to be. We sat and talked and then ended up laughing and joking and agreed that I could end up with a better figure after it was all done!

A further appointment had been made for me to see the Surgeon on Wednesday 10th September and to be honest we all just felt that until we had it confirmed by Mr Bristol that this was the final outcome, we all just went about our business.

My son and his wife and daughter had flown to Spain on Friday 29th August and I could not see any point in ringing them until I had been told the news for definite but on Wednesday 10th September I went to see Mr Bristol, who confirmed that it was a cancerous breast tumour in the right breast and micro-calcifications in the left which could in time turn cancerous - but that owing to the fact that they had caught it so early there was a 98.9% chance that the cancer would not have spread and that after surgery I would be in the clear - but as he informed me he was not God and nothing could be that certain.

From that moment on - as far I was concerned it was now certain I had cancer and I was not going to let this pull me down - I was going to keep strong not only for myself but for my family and I knew if I could have positive and not negative thoughts I was going to get through this.

Mr Bristol (the Breast Surgeon) could not believe it - as his words to me were "Chris where has this suddenly appeared from" as three months previous there was nothing there. He went into a full explanation of what would happen and tried to reassure me that everything would be all right - and I turned to him and said "as long as you make me look like Katie Price and not Kenny Everett, I should be ok". That broke the ice for us and then things really started to move. Before we even left the Hospital that night I was having my Questionnaire read to me and a Consent Form to sign - things were moving and moving fast.

I told my work colleagues the next day (there was a few tears that day - they were all so sweet) but I don't think any of them could understand why I was not breaking down - no point is there - what would it achieve.

On Friday 12th September I had to go to the Hospital (my daughter came with me) I was to have an E.C.G. and an X-Ray to check the chest area and I was supposed to have had photos taken ready for the reconstruction - but unfortunately the photographer was not there that day. Everything seemed to be ok and they made me an appointment to go in on Saturday 13th September to have the Sentinel Lymph Glands Biopsy done. This was to check that the cancer had not spread. It was all moving really quickly.

My main concern when I got home on the Friday morning, was that I knew I had to break the news to my son who had just returned from holiday that morning - I was dreading that more than anything. That was my second time of having a few tears - he just seemed speechless - so he spoke to my daughter who explained a few things and bless his heart he drove up from Bristol in the pouring rain just to see me - he is 31 years old and that was the first time he had ever bought me flowers!!! I knew then that he was concerned and he loved me!

We sat and spoke and discussed it all and we all said again that we have got to have a positive approach and we will all get through it together.

CHAPTER 3

Keith took me to the Hospital on Saturday morning and bless his heart he looked really down but he told me that he was not actually feeling very well himself. So I told him to come on home as I would just read and wait for them to take me to Theatre.

My daughter had not bought me flowers - she had bought me a bottle of my favourite Eternity perfume - which I took with me still boxed up in my over night bag and I just kept thinking of Steve's flowers and Nicki's perfume.

Sure enough - not much time went by until I was given the Designer backless gown and the lovely non-colour-co-ordinated tights - very fetching - all I had to do now was to wait for my limo to take me to the Theatre - I only hoped we were not going to see "The Fallen Madonna with the Big Boobies" but to be honest - by the time the anaesthetist patted my hand twice I was not awake to see or feel anything!

I came round about 4.00 and was taken back to my room - absolutely gasping for a cup of tea as I had not eaten or drunk anything since 7.30 that morning. I was put in a side ward on my own - which was nice - purely because I had to be monitored every two hours and it would not have been fair on the other patients, some of whom I had met throughout the day walking passed to go to the loo - when you think we are all in the same predicament it makes life a little easier - just because I am having a double mastectomy does not make it any harder or easier for those that are having one.

Keith came into see me at 6.00 but again was not looking too good and saying he did not feel too well, so again I asked him to go home at 7.00 so that he could get some rest, as when I came out the next day I would need him there. I was not the best person to be sat with I suppose as I looked a bit like a Smurf - as they inject you with a blue dye and it obviously comes out in your face and your wee (I had wasted money buying loo blues for the toilet)

All the staff were so helpful and friendly so at least when I go in for the major operation, at least I will already know some of them.

Keith picked me up the next morning at 10.00 and to me he seemed very distant - we got home and he made me a cup of tea but instead of sitting with me he was pottering about in the garden and I was trying to talk to him - I decided at that point that I would go to bed at 11.00 as I had not had much rest the night before and he said that he would go out shopping. I could not sleep so I got up at 12.00 and Keith was obviously still out but he had left his mobile on the side - he would never ever have done that normally as he always says (even during a normal day if he is going out without me somewhere) just ring me if you need me. I was now getting quite concerned - because I felt as though I was dealing with this in the best way that I could - but he - maybe along with quite a few other men in the same situation - could not come to terms with it. So I text my daughter to ask if Keith had said anything to her - but she told me no.

I did confront Keith when he came home and he looked most upset that I had even had those thoughts - he said that it was me as a person that he loved and that he would support me 100% through this - that made me feel an awful lot better - what a relief.

Nicki - my daughter - could not settle so she decided that she would come up that evening and stayed over. She worked from here on the Monday and her work have been absolutely fantastic telling her that I come first. My work have been fantastic as well - I cannot believe how understanding people can be and are there to support me.

My daughter is coming back up tonight (Tuesday 16th September) and staying with me tomorrow - making sure that I eat and drink healthily and my son is coming up on Thursday to do what he can and my daughter in law is coming up on Friday - I have not had the major operation yet and everyone is being so supportive.

My journey has only just started and I am going to proceed with this book along my journey - even if you do not want to read it - it is a good therapy for me.

CHAPTER 4

I have got to go back to the Clinic on Wednesday 24th September to get my results of the biopsies (and I hope they are going to be clear) and to also have the photos done - I am hoping on that day I will get a date for the operation and I just hope that it will be in October as they have told me that it will be about three months for me to be fit again - and it is my grand-daughters 1st Birthday on the 23rd January 2009 and I want to be there to be able to hold her and to see her blow out the candle on her cake - and I will be there and I will do that. I am not going to treat it as though it is a major operation, I am going to treat it more as an "Extreme Body Makeover" for her first birthday.

The wounds under the arms today (Tuesday 16th) are feeling not too bad and I am doing my exercises three times a day. I will use this book almost as a diary to assist me on remembering what happened on what day.

It has also just occurred to me that we have not yet had time to even pick out and order our Wedding Photos - things have happened that quickly. I have also had to cancel our holiday that was booked for the 26th to Bulgaria and the taxi that was to take us to the airport but never mind - we will have that holiday even if not this year. The same old story though isn't it - you put a claim in to the Insurance Company and it is the same old delay tactics but I did get paid out eventually.

I have been sat on my own today and you just keep thinking that life all around you still goes on – because unless it is something that affects you personally then life for other people does still continue as normal.

We have lived in the house now for just over three years and the couple two doors down - who unfortunately we had a few words with a couple of years ago - Peg (the wife) called round today - gave me a hug and a kiss and bought me a lovely plant and a beautiful card and said that if there was anything at all I needed or wanted I just had to ask and bless her all the way through she has called up to see me with different gifts.

It is such a shame that we all live in a world that is crumbling around us but when someone has a crisis in their life you realise that friends, family and neighbours will actually rally round to help - it really could be a wonderful world if people would stop having so much hatred and being so greedy.

It is now Thursday and I must admit I feel really well - the stitches have stopped itching and the wounds seem to be feeling quite comfortable. To be honest unless I take my top off and see the blue coverings on the wounds, I really don't feel as though anything has been done at all. I am bright and cheerful and have not felt as well as this for a long time. Lets just hope it continues.

CHAPTER 5

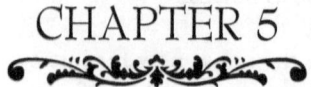

Well I have been at home for a week now and returned to work yesterday. It is not until you return to work that you realise how relaxing and how well you feel when you are at home and I must admit by the time I got home on the first day I was feeling really tired. Having said that it was nice to have had the week before and having visitors coming to see me - different ones every day and everyone being so cheerful - it made me feel a lot brighter and fitter in myself. So thank you to all those visitors that I had that week (and they know who they are). It was not only me going through a traumatic period but Keith as well and he also needed some support.

You also come to terms with the fact that the people who annoy you or have upset you in some way are really quite irrelevant and you just feel to yourself that your life is not worth even considering those people - again I am not going to name or shame but if you do happen to read this book, you will know who you are!

Under my arms ache just a little but there again I am a Receptionist and the constant answering the phone did not help the situation - but my lovely friends at work have got me a headset (don't think I will look like Madonna but lets hope it does the trick).

I can honestly say though that since I had the operation to remove the lymph nodes it was not as bad as I was expecting it to be - I think the worst part is when they started to itch a little and you knew that you could not scratch them - but other than that, there were times that I had forgotten I had even had it done. It was only when I got undressed in the evening and saw the dressings that it all came back.

I have to go to the Hospital tomorrow to have the dressings removed (even though both breasts still have the blue dye on them - they are fading but it wont wash off) and to get the results of the biopsies. I also have to have the reconstruction photos taken and hopefully a date for the operation. I really just want to get tomorrow out of the way so that I can start to plan my life.

My husband is acting as normal as possible - and letting me do things because I feel so well I think - for me continuing to cook the dinner - do the ironing - the vacuuming - making the bed - putting the rubbish out - I think our partners just get so used to us doing these things that they just switch off - we only have ourselves to blame don't we? Having said that - if I had not been able to do it then I just could not have done it - I sometimes wonder if by pushing yourself just that little bit without overdoing it - maybe it does assist with a speedy recovery. It is only when you know that you have a partner to help you if you need it - that you realise that there must be so many people out there going through the same traumatic time and that they have no friends or family at all to help them through this - puts your moaning in perspective I think.

Well I returned to work this week - but had my appointment at the Breast Cancer Clinic on Wednesday 24th September - unfortunately I did not receive the news that I was expecting - did not feel upset or angry just a bit deflated.

Apparently the biopsies on the left side were clear but the biopsies on the right showed that the cancer had spread into some of the lymph glands. This then meant I had some choices to make. I could either have the double mastectomy and have the left side reconstructed at the same time - I could have the double mastectomy and not have any reconstruction at this time - and the reason they could not do the reconstruction on the right was because I was going to need chemotherapy and radiotherapy to try and zap the cancer before the surgeon would do the reconstruction this side.

I was more deflated than anything because I was convinced, having spoken to the Surgeon earlier that he was 98.9% certain that the cancer was contained and therefore when I was admitted to hospital I could have the double mastectomy and the double reconstruction at the same time and the fact that the cancer was contained, I would not require to have radiotherapy or chemotherapy!

I did have the photographs taken for the reconstruction (just in case) and that was quite a pleasant experience - beautiful photo studio and a lovely young lady taking the pictures.

I came home with my head spinning to be honest - I was quite happy with the wounds (after having had the dressings removed that day as well) and all seemed to be fine but I now had the big decision to make. The only thing would be if I had the double mastectomy and one reconstruction - then I would have a bra with just one prosthesis which could be more awkward than having a bra containing two. The other decision would then have to be made that if after a year -

would I really feel like going through the whole thing again and a further three months of torture?

My daughter returned to us from Nottingham that night and we just spoke and discussed everything, but as we all agreed, it was best to have a word with the surgeon next time I saw him.

I go to see the surgeon again on Wednesday 1st October and they hope to take me in a few days after that.

Obviously we phoned friends and family to tell them the latest update and one very dear friend of mine (Ellen) informed me that one of her friends had gone through the mastectomy and the reconstruction, which took approximately nine hours of surgery and she told Ellen that if she were me, knowing what she knew, she would just have the mastectomy and forget about the reconstruction.

I mean really in all honesty - I am nearly 60 - I think my days of Kylie Minogue cut-through the front dresses and the topless sunbathing on the beach are over for me anyway - even if I did not need any surgery at all.

Also, if you think about it - there are probably only two people who are going to see me naked, one is me and one is my husband - and he has truthfully told me that as long as I am healthy and free of cancer he does not mind what I look like undressed (I think he may change his mind on that one when I go from a Dolly Parton to an Arnie Schwarzenegger!!!)

I am back into work this morning and I now have to tell all my work colleagues that unfortunately I did not receive the news that I thought I was going to get. This is part of the hard bit - the telling to people who genuinely care.

It is now Thursday the 2nd October and I am just about heading out the front door to go to work - but I had to put my thoughts down before I went.

CHAPTER 6

Yesterday my daughter and I spent the day together - we had a lovely girlie day - going shopping and then chilling by watching Sex and the City DVD - lovely - made us laugh (and a few tears as well) - but great film. We then had our trip up to the Breast Clinic to have the final talk with the Surgeon - but unfortunately - as usual - it was a three hour delay before we got into see him - but the staff are so dedicated and work such long hours - and again it puts it in perspective when you see so many ladies going in to see him and although we all have the same problem - every one of us is an individual.

We all went armed with our bombardment of questions - but in all fairness Mr Bristol was so lovely and explained everything fully that we have decided against any reconstruction at this stage (just to be on the safe side that once the mastectomy on the right side has been done) we want to ensure that there is no cancer - or very little cancer there. I will not find that out for about ten days after the operation.

If it turns out that there is none or very little cancer it will mean that I will not need chemotherapy or radiotherapy and I will just have to take a tablet every day for the rest of my life to ensure that the cancer does not return. If it looks as though I have a minimum amount of cancer there - then I may only need a few doses of radiotherapy.

I did tell Mr Bristol that I may consider the reconstruction after the mastectomy and the light at the end of the tunnel is that if there is no cancer - or very little - there is no reason why I cannot have the reconstruction within the next few months!

I am still keeping very cheerful and taking care of myself by not trying to overdo it and I do feel remarkably well in myself.

The scars under the arms now from the Lymph Node operation are clearing exceptionally well and I have had no horrible side effects following that operation. So should you or anyone you know, ever need that operation done, please do not worry - it is a walk in the park!!

I will continue with my story once I have been into Hospital - which is now scheduled for Saturday 11th October - so as soon as I return home - I will once again give you my thoughts and experiences of going through that major double mastectomy. Forever thinking and keeping positive and I know my mum is looking over me at all times and taking good care of me.

It is now Friday 10th and I go into Hospital tomorrow at 8.00 - been quite a funny week really - still seems to me as though it is happening to someone else and I am looking at it happening.

Everyone at work has been absolutely great - we have all had a laugh and a joke - even one of the guys (John) bought a badge called The Boob Inspector" as he thought it would be advisable if he inspected the "before and after" - in your dreams baby!!!

I was also a little bit tearful on Wednesday night when I went to bed - I don't know why and for no apparent reason I just saw this picture of myself undressed and I looked awful - my body looked disgusting and mutilated and after having shed a lot of tears and a few sobs and managed to get out "I am going to look so horrible" I then got over it again and settled off down to sleep.

My daughter spent the day with me today and we had a lovely girlie day - I had a manicure (but obviously without the nail varnish) as you are not allowed any makeup etc in hospital and she had the back massage - then we did some down town things and some shoppie things - came home and had a nice bowl of fresh soup and a fresh roll and off she went again to Bristol.

I am really confident about tomorrow and I trust everyone that will be "working on me" with my life and I know that once the operation is done and I am out of recovery and back to the ward - then we have gone that one small step (the first of many to come I can imagine) but at least we have made it. What makes me even more confident is that I believe my mum is looking after me - had quite a few signs now (but they would only be personal to me) but when Nicki and I came back from shopping today - there lying in my drive was a white feather! And that is what clinched it for me and all I can say is "Thanks Mum".

My dad travelled up North having come to stay on the Tuesday and I am sure that once he actually saw me and realised that I was in a very good space he was able to travel up to see his family without worrying about me too much. I would just at this stage (now that it is all over) like to say a big thank you to my dad - it was a terrible time for him and having to cope with it all on his own and I really appreciate all his help and concern through the terrible ordeal.

Some of my friends and family have taken it harder than others - but I think that is what makes us all individuals. But I cannot begin to thank all those people that have been so kind in sending me cards - emails - text messages and phone calls and everyone that has spoken to me has wished me all the very best - even my Managing Director at work made that special phone call to me on his day off - all of these things just give you that extra shove that you need because all those people are genuine and that you know that everyone really loves you for you (not your body)!

I am sorry that I have not been able to see my little grand-daughter before I went in - but they all had nasty colds and that was the last thing I wanted - but I know I am going to see a lot more of her in the days - weeks and years to come.

My case is now packed and I am just waiting for my husband to come home so that we can have a nice cosy meal and a nice cosy evening together - all ready to be up at 6.00 am to be at the Hospital for 8.00am - not really the same as getting up to go on holiday at that time in the morning with your cases packed - but it is certainly a journey that I have never been on before.

I will carry on with my story once I have returned from hospital as I intend to keep a diary of events of the days that I am in there.

There is only one other thing that bothers me – not as much as the operation, but have you ever been in a Waiting Room (like the one I was in whilst waiting to have the Sentinel Lymph Gland operation) and you come across the most annoying person you have met for a long time - the one that never seems to stop moaning about everything! This is the person having a lump removed (and not interested at all in what other people are going through). She is the one that you are dreading having in the bed next to you in the ward for the next 5-10 days - oh well fingers crossed that if she is the curtains can be pulled at all times of the day!! Again - I will keep you posted on that one.

Keith and I arrived at the Hospital at 7.30 on Saturday 11th but unfortunately did not get a bed until 11.30 and I did not go down for surgery until 2.00 - everything seemed to go extremely well and I was sitting up in bed by 6.00 waiting for Keith to arrive for visiting.

On Sunday 12th I was feeling really well - the only things that I did not like were the three drains coming from my body especially the one under the right arm which was draining the lymph glands part - that was really uncomfortable - felt like a red hot Stanley knife cutting me when I moved. Nicki and Keith came into visit at 3.00 and I was very tearful - I think partly to do with the anaesthetic and the morphine and partly because I was so uncomfortable.

I did feel so sorry for Nicki though - she offered to help me go to the toilet as it was quite awkward with the three drains and trying to lift your gown at the same time - you just then realise how vulnerable we all can be at times - I never thought I would get to the stage where my own daughter had to take me to the loo! I thought as well it may have been nice to have a designer bag to hold the bottles, but they only give you a pillowcase!

I did have a bit of a problem later on as I went to the toilet and pulled out one of the drains - not very clever. Also in the evening when it was quite late - again I went to the toilet and ended up with all gunk running down me - it appeared that because the nurses had not checked the drainage bottles - one of mine (the main one!) had got over-full and the bottle could just not hold any more and it blew the vacuum - so at 9.30

at night I was being cleaned up and fresh bottles being put in place. Did not have too bad a night.

On Monday 13th I had one of the drains taken out and I was asked by the doctors if I was doing my exercises and I just told them that it was so painful with the drain there - they said that it had to stay and I had to do them. No sympathy vote there then!

Tuesday 14th - had an absolutely awful night - we had an elderly Irish woman suffering with dementia and she kept us all awake all night as she kept holding a two way conversation with herself - we were all at screaming pitch by the morning. Also a lot of activity going on through the night.

At least I had Jan – who was the lady in the bed next to me and we became good friends - we still keep in touch now – we had a few laughs (case of having to!)

I had my dressings changed - everything looking good and I felt so much more comfortable - the stinging had almost stopped and I really pushed forward to get my exercises done - I just wanted to get out and get home and the Doctor had told me that I would not be out until at least Friday or Saturday - how depressing.

Wednesday 15th - another awful night - I did not feel particularly well but the nurse did not seem to be overly concerned - I just sat and cried and asked my mum to "please get me out of here". In the morning the Doctors did their rounds - I had oozed all I had to ooze - the wound was looking good and I got my Discharge Papers and I left at 12.00 that day - felt awful as Jan was in tears as she said she could not do this without me - I told her that I would phone and text her and if she ever needed me to give me a call.

CHAPTER 7

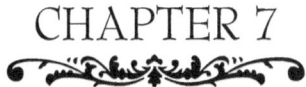

Thursday 16ᵗʰ - it had been such a relief to get home last night - and I must admit I was extremely tearful but Keith , Nicki and Steve made me feel positive again - and it was so lovely to have a bath and freshen up - you just had this awful smell about you. Did not have too bad a night - but did not sleep as well as I thought - got up - beautiful day - the sun was shining and it was just so fantastic to be alive and really not to be in any pain at all.

The Hospital experience was one thing and some of the people I met were something else.

None of us were really over enamoured with the cleanliness in the place - we used to get up to go to the bathroom and there would be pots of urine just lying on the floor and the window sills waiting to be collected and they could remain there for hours.

Jan (the girl mentioned previously) was in such a state because she had to have a blood transfusion and we said that we would get her through it and help as much as we could. That evening a cat came onto the ward and into the office - I cannot believe what a fuss and commotion was made by the nurses over this cat - just put the bloody thing outside on the road. Jan's blood arrived at the office and the cat was still sitting in there!! When the nurse eventually came with the blood to Jan's bed - I said "excuse me - you are surely not going to give her that blood when you have had it in the office with a cat in there" - this nurse really had attitude and I was seriously thinking of reporting her to the Medical Board - her attitude was absolutely disgusting. Another lovely lady - Maggie - she had leaked out of her drains and she was lying in her urine bed-soaked sheets and covers for over two hours! Called to see Maggie on Friday 12th June to be told she had passed away six weeks previous - Jan and I were so upset as we wanted to take her out for a meal. I just hope she is out of pain and at peace now bless her.

We cannot blame the nurses - they are so rushed off their feet and some of them could not do enough for you - others just seemed to give off an aura that they did not want to be in nursing but at least it was a job.

Having said that - we all had a bit of a laugh and we all kept each others spirits up.

My next journey is Wednesday 22nd when I have to return to the hospital to have my staples removed and to be told if I have or have not got any more cancer! Still thinking positive and I am sure we will get through this without too much hassle - that is my theory at the moment.

All I can say about the double mastectomy is - that it really was not as horrendous an operation that I thought it would be – bearing in mind I was a 38C when I went in and a nothing when I came out - which is quite a shock to the system. I haven't at this stage actually seen the wound as I am wrapped up in a water-proof bandage.

I am not quite sure on the feelings of Keith at this stage - he did help me get undressed and he did help me get into the bath and he was extremely quiet - said he was very tired.

I was very tearful on the Wednesday evening and Keith was there to cuddle me but on the Thursday we watched a programme called The Lion Man and one of the baby lions had died and they held a ceremony for him before they buried him and Keith was in floods of tears - I think that was just the excuse he was looking for.

I don't think for one minute he despises the way I look - he is not that sort - and it just still seems very strange that I do not have this weight to carry around - in fact I lost nine pounds in weight whilst in hospital and I am convinced that eight of those were from my boobs!

It is now Friday afternoon and my daughter has been with me all day - again had a girlie day and did a bit of shopping but I realise now how tired I get and you just cant do it - so we came home - had some lunch - and she did my nails for me - she then decided to go so that I could have a sleep before Keith came home - but I just wanted to get on with my book whilst I was in the mood.

Some lovely bouquets of flowers arrived today - some completely unexpected and a real surprise and I would like to thank those of you who sent me them – they cheered me up no end – after having a few tears on their arrival!

I have been out of hospital nearly five days now and the time just seems to be flying by - I am still feeling really well but will be glad when the dressings and the staples are out as I feel they are restricting me in what I can do and what I can wear.

My daughter told me how beautiful I looked and my son told me he had never seen me looking so good - in fact I looked ten years younger - and that really meant a lot to me.

My husband on the other hand - I am not sure - he does not seem to be making any comments at all - will help me when I ask him - but has not once said that I am looking good or I am looking nice in what I am wearing - but maybe this is his way of dealing with it and I am going to give him the space that he needs. He may be opening up to some of the lads at work and if that is his way - then so be it.

It was our anniversary yesterday (3 months) and what a three months this has been - but we went and collected our wedding photos and stopped at the Rising Sun and had a lovely Sunday meal - it was nice to be able to be out to be able to celebrate.

I heard from Jan at the weekend to say that she was now out - and I felt so pleased for her - I am thinking of the other ladies that were in hospital with me but as I have said before Jan and I seemed to bond together and I am really interested to see how she progresses.

It was my first day of being home today on my own - it was quite nice really - did not wake until about 10.00 and then just had an easy day - writing letters- sorting photos - sending emails and just sorting general rubbish.

Have decided that the rest of my body is also going to need toning up a bit so once I have been to the hospital on Wednesday I will be able to ask what form of exercise - other than my arms - I can do. I did take myself for a little walk down the road and back this morning and it was so lovely to get out in the fresh air.

I know that once you have had the lymph glands removed you have to be very careful about lots of things - so again when I see the surgeon on Wednesday I will just clarify a few points.

I am still staying positive for Wednesday and will be so pleased if he turns to me and says "you are in the clear Chris - we have got it all" - what a wonderful moment that will be - so keeping everything crossed - and praying to my mum to help me on the next step - it is one other day that will be nice to put behind me.

Well it is now Friday 24th - I could not face writing any part of the book yesterday.

Went to Hospital for a 3.25 appointment and got in just after 5.00 - the Breast Cancer nurse looked at the wound (must say I am taking on the appearance of a pyjama case now) and she said that everything looked fine and so continued with removing all the staples - not too bad an experience really - just had a few hot flushes and a few ouches but really it was quite painless" - it was nice to have Nicki and Keith in with me.

The surgeon then came in and looked and prodded and said that yes everything was fine the surgery had gone remarkably well and the wound was looking really good and healing well - and no I did not have to do anything more to the wound just to let it heal in its own time.

Yes the cancer completely gone in the left breast and the tumour removed from the right - but they had taken 22 lymph nodes out at the same time and two of them were cancerous - hooray I thought - that is it - I am just going to have to take the one tablet a day. No! It did not seem as though that was going to be the case at all.

I could either just take the tablet - which would give me a 76% chance. I could take the tablet and the radiotherapy - which would give me an 82% chance or I could have the chemotherapy - radiotherapy and the tablet and that would give me an 86% chance BUT if having taken any of these options it could be that I would be clear of cancer BUT I could be involved in a serious road accident - or die of a heart attack etc!! Oh help!! My head was spinning.

My daughter and my husband were with me the whole time and I did try and look at them both when the plaster was removed and I must admit I did not see any immediate shock in their faces - that helped a lot.

My husband held my hand all the time the staples were being removed and that helped a great deal too.

They told me not to make any instant decisions - as the surgeon wanted to have a second meeting with the Medical Team as he had not been in the meeting on the Tuesday and he was questioning some of the notes - makes you feel really confident doesn't it?

By the time I was being bombarded with the removal of the staples - the Surgeon and the Breast Care Nurse I could not take any more and as we walked out the Hospital I broke down - I just felt as though my body had been completely mutilated and I still needed further treatment - why - I only had TWO cancerous lymph nodes!! Surely this was good news wasn't it??

My daughter told me I had not gone backwards - basically I had been given the ALL CLEAR but just as a PRECAUTION I was being offered the after care service - I DID NOT need to take any of it if I did not want to - it was not as if they had said - we are sorry the cancer has spread through your body and if you don't have these treatments you will be dead in six months time - then I felt better and we went out for a meal and I had a few glasses of wine and felt much better after that.

I got home but could not settle in bed - the staple removal was actually a bit tender and it just seemed as though I could not get comfortable - so once again I headed off to the spare room - bad mistake - I just had everything going round and round in my head and yes I am going to admit it - I did cry myself to sleep.

I woke up in the morning - looked at the scar - thought - you look all right babe - you are going to do this - you have got this far and you will go the distance. Don't worry about making any decisions as after the meeting of Tuesday you may find that they all agree that you do not need the chemo or the radio therapy and you only need the tablet - so you have woken up for another morning - you are feeling really well in yourself so live for today and let each day takes its course - when you get the results from the meeting - then make your decision - but only after you have talked it through with an oncologist - they know what they are talking about and they can tell you what the advantages are and what the side effects may be.

So I busied myself around the house - I put some washing on and hung it out - I made myself some lunch - sat down and watched my afternoon programmes - went up and had a shower and washed my hair (really chuffed that I can do all these things for myself) did my exercises by which time Keith had come home from work - we sat and chatted - had a drink - cooked the meal together and the evening came and went with no real discussions about what decision we were going to make.

Anyway I am feeling really well again this morning - always feel a bit tight across the chest after I have woken up and a little sore under the arms (but that is only the sores caused by the bandage that will soon heal) - so I am now going off to do my exercises and have a cup of coffee.

I will continue this now probably on Thursday - as the meeting is on the Tuesday but the nurse cannot ring me until the Thursday - so let us just enjoy life to the full until then eh!

On the 22nd October I had a meeting with my surgeon who explained that all on the left was clear and they had got all the cancer from the right - but because it had gone into the lymph glands it was suggested that I had chemotherapy - radiotherapy and tamoxifen - but to go away and think about it.

My head was in a turmoil - what is it about the two "C" words - cancer and chemotherapy!

On Tuesday 28th October I had an appointment to see the Oncologist at 5.00 - once again my daughter came up - awful night - sleeting and windy.

At 4.00 I received a telephone call from Jane at the Breast Cancer Clinic to say "Hello Christina - so when do we next see you again" I told her that I was not sure as I had to go and see the Consultant at 5.00. She said yes she knew and they were going to discuss my radiotherapy treatment - but I said that I thought I had to have chemo first - she said no - she had my notes in front of her and it was only radiotherapy that I needed not the chemo - I was so ecstatic - I was crying with joy when Keith walked through the door - I explained what had happened and he said that we would have a glass of champers when we got home.

When my daughter arrived and we told her - she just had that look on her face and she said "I am sorry mum I just don't believe it"

Well we got to the Oncology Department - once again had to wait about two hours before we got in - and the first thing the Consultant said was that I had had everything explained so we best discuss when the first course of chemotherapy would start! What!!! I told him "I don't need it" and explained about the phone call that I had - he was most taken aback and said that he did not know where she had got this information from because it was a yes - I did need chemotherapy and yes I would lose my hair (which was the next question I had asked him) and so you can imagine I just burst into tears - I could not believe it - I was so angry - so the next morning I phoned up the Breast Cancer Clinic and gave them a good telling off.

They did ring me back and explained what had happened - but it really is not good enough - and also they had had a very strong message left by the Consultant the night before.

So yes - I have decided to give myself the best possible chance and today Monday 3rd November I go and see the Breast Cancer Nurse to sort out my prosthesis and then I travel down to see the Chemotherapy Nurse who is going to give me a pre-chemo chat.

I then go Tuesday 4th November at 9.30 to have my first chemotherapy - not looking forward to it one little bit, but just keep assuring myself that it cannot be that bad!!!

On Saturday I chose a wig from the internet - took the picture into the hairdresser and she cut my hair to match the wig - looks really nice I think - so that if I do start to lose my hair I have got my wig on standby. Your hair does start to fall out in handfuls - you find it all over the pillows and the cushions and it is quite distressing - as the weeks have gone on the hair is still coming out and is very very thin (I am just passed my 5th chemo) - but at the end of the day you know that it will grow back.

I feel at the moment that most of my body is sitting on the bedside cabinet - my boobs are pinned into my bra (that is the cumfys) so they don't ride up and out whilst I am out and about and shortly my hair will be sitting looking at me as well - I cant read a thing without my glasses - which sit alongside the boobs - the only thing I hope do not let me down at this time are my teeth - I hardly need them looking at me from a glass also on the bedside table - I think we may have to get some bigger bedside furniture.

Anyway to top that I called in to have a coffee with all my workmates on the Wednesday - was given my pay cheque - brilliant they had paid me my full pay for the whole month - I was so chuffed.

At 6.00 that night I had a phone call from one of the girls to say that they had all been called in at 5.00 - given their pay cheques and a letter and all told not to report for work the next day as the company had gone into liquidation! So not only had I lost my boobs I had lost my job as well!

Decided on Saturday morning to go to the Job Centre to sign on - it is closed on a Saturday!! Decided to call into Marks and Spencer to get a prosthesis bra ready for Monday morning (they don't sell them in Cheltenham I have to go to Bristol) great! I am still trying to fight to get my travel insurance to pay out for my cancelled holiday - so at the moment - it does not seem as though lady luck is looking down on me - but I just keep telling myself - I am still alive - I have a wonderful husband and family and friends who are all there to support me - and there are people out there a lot worse off than me.

So once again - pick yourself up - dust yourself off and get ready to take another week of challenges.

On Monday 3rd November I had to go to the Breast Clinic to be measured for my prosthesis - "measured" - you take your bra in - they tell you that you that you are a size 6 (or whatever bust size you are) they give you the prosthesis to put in your bra and off you go!!!

I then had to go and see the Pre Chemo Nurse who explained all the treatment and the nasty side effects etc etc - they then take a blood test to make sure that you are fit and well enough to have the chemo the next day - well you come out of there and your head is spinning - you are so worried about all these terrible side effects that you feel sick and nauseas before you start.

CHAPTER 8

My daughter came up that evening as she was coming with me. We got up at 6.30 Tuesday morning and we were at the hospital at 9.15 - one good thing about chemo (if there is a good thing) at least you get a Parking Permit which really does help as apparently you can be there at 9.30 in the morning and not be walking out until about 10.00 at night (so I was told by some patients).

My appointment was at 9.30 and once again by 10.45 no one had called us, so twice my daughter had to go up to Reception to find out how long we had to wait to see the Doctor - it appeared as though when I booked in at the Chemo Reception they had not passed on my Blue Form to the Radiotherapy Section (which was where we had to wait) - strangely not long after that we were called into see the Consultant - it has now gone 11.00 - all I had to do was sign a Consent Form (could I not have done that the day before with the Nurse) - he then asked the nurse how long we would have to wait and she said we would not be seen before 4.00 so if we would like to leave a mobile number they would ring us when they were ready and we had to be back within about 15 to 20 minutes - no problem we said we would be back by 3.00. We decided to go and get some food shopping and then go back home for lunch - would give us plenty of time.

No - did not work out that way - walking around filling our trolley - it is now 12.00 and we have not been left the hospital that long - and it is Brian from Oncology saying that my treatment is ready!!! What!! When you sit there waiting you are there for about four hours when you leave you have 15 to 20 minutes to get back!! So we rushed our shopping through - rushed back to the hospital - were there at 12.20 - at 1.00 we are still waiting - so my daughter once again had to go to Reception to say that we were called back and we were still waiting!! The receptionist went off and said that they were waiting for a spare chair and an available nurse in the downstairs room. At 1.15 my name was called and we had to go to the upstairs room!

We were met by a fantastic Oncologist called Brian who really made my daughter and I feel at ease straight away - and by the time they have got the saline drip fixed - put your hand in hot water to try and get a vein - sorted all the syringes out - then fitted the canular to your hand and away you go - we started at 1.30 and were walking out at 2.30 - but I just hope I can have Brian everytime - he was absolutely fantastic - and I had no funny effects when they were administering the drugs which apparently is a good sign - just a little twinge in the nose (which apparently is supposed to happen).

We came home I felt fine - had something to eat - my daughter left having looked absolutely shattered. I think she felt as bewildered and scared as me and I will at this point say that I was absolutely terrified (after having not slept at all the previous night wondering what awful things were going to happen to me that day).

I kept thinking all night that something was going to happen - sweating - vomiting - headache - sore throat etc etc and by 6.00 when the alarm went off I was still wide awake and kept thinking that it would kick in throughout the morning.

I got up and dressed and went into town and bought a few things that I thought I might need - for example a couple of turbans (for when my hair falls out) some Velcro rollers as you cannot use hairdryers - curling tongs etc - and I ordered a couple of prosthesis bras (and again what a lovely lady that looked after me) owns a tiny little lingerie shop in Cheltenham and she was an absolute star.

Came home and felt a bit tired so went to bed at 1.00 and slept till 3.00 (apart from the quick phone call my daughter made to me at 2.00) - got up prepared and cooked the meal but by 9.00 that night I was tired. I have now made an appointment for Monday 10th November as you have to have a flu jab (highly recommended) as apparently your immune system goes to rock bottom. I have my next chemotherapy session on the 25th November but that depends on whether your blood count is high enough.

My daughter is coming up to spend the evening with me and all day tomorrow as she is flying off to Cancun on Monday - so as I still feel all right this morning I am going to do a little food shopping trip to Sainsbury's and will then return and probably head off to bed for a few hours - because although it is quite good to keep yourself a bit active - it is also better if you can rest and give your body a chance. So for now - I have everything crossed that it continues this way - probably wont but that is where positive thinking comes in - so next time there is something to report I will hit the keyboard again - I just thank the Lord every day that I wake up that I have in fact woken up and nothing is seriously wrong - that has got to be to do with the positive thinking.

It is now Monday and I should have had Ellen come to stay (10th November) but unfortunately due to the awful weather we decided to knock it on the head. I even cancelled my flu jab and re-scheduled for tomorrow.

I must say I was a little bit tearful on Friday when I was shopping with my daughter and that passed - then yesterday - Sunday I was even more tearful and I also had a bout of the runs - but fortunately it did not last - I think we were to blame for that as we had gone all day without anything to eat and then had a great big Sunday roast!!!

As I am now unable to work for quite a few months I have decided to contact Social Security to try and get some sort of benefit as I have also lost my job - and as I have never claimed for anything in my life I think it is about time I reaped some of the benefits!

It is Tuesday 11th November and when I woke up this morning I felt I had been hit by a bus - just could not be bothered to get out of bed at 6.00 when Keith got up for breakfast. Just stayed in bed and slept - woke about 10.00 and felt a bit better. It is now 1.30 and I still feel as though something big has run into me - but I am going to have a bath and get dressed as I must go and get my flu jab today - really need that on top of everything else.

Oh well - there is no point in moaning - at least I am at home and can do what I like when I like - it could be worse I could be in a hospital bed rigged up to drips and things - so once again - stop feeling sorry for yourself - you are alive - you are not in pain so keep on this positive thinking.

Well Tuesday 11th I went for my flu jab - what a palaver that was as well - first of all they said they did not think I could have it I whilst under-going chemotherapy - but I told them that it was the Consultant who told me I HAD to have it and as soon as possible - then they said they would have to have written authority from my own doctor - and I told them that I had spoken to my doctor that morning and I told her that I was going for the flu jab that day - she did not say anything about not being able to have one - then they tried to find some sort of Official Form on the computer - which they could not find - then the nurse got another doctor involved - and I just suggested that why did they not ring the Chemotherapy Help Line as that is what it was there for - which eventually they decided to do and they were given permission for me to receive the jab - hooray - I could have contracted flu in the amount of time I was sat there waiting - but I then had to advise them that I could not have the needle in the arm due to the surgery that I had had - they had to then consult a book to see where abouts on my body I could have it - so if it is any help to any of you out there who have to go through the same rigmarole as me you can say - yes you know for a fact that you can have the flu jab during the treatment of chemotherapy and it does not matter how far into the treatment you are and yes (if you have had the lymph glands removed also) that they stick the needle in the top of your thigh - there all done and dusted and over in about twenty seconds. Mind, I have to say - that I am quite relieved that they did look thoroughly into it - as they may have been right and I could have ended up being a bit ippy dippy - or a bit more than I feel usually! You also have to remember that if you have blood pressure taken it cannot be done on the arm it has to be done on the calf.

I am going to say at this stage in the book also that I must just thank everyone close to me for being there - my daughter who has just been absolutely brilliant and if she has been scared or worried at any stage during this time has never ever let me know or never ever let it show and can I say a big thank you to all her very close friends and colleagues who have also got her through this terrible time - my son (who although has not rushed about everywhere as there has been no need) has given me words of comfort on the phone (as has his wife Becci) and he has obviously taken it very much to heart, which I am sure is one of the reasons that he has not been feeling well himself lately also to Becci's parents who have constantly enquired as to my well-being   - my husband who although has remained very quiet - all through this trauma has still been there for me with a kiss and a cuddle and a big shoulder to cry on when I have my off days - my dad who has tried to stay out of the way in order to help but as like my daughter - because he is on his own and has to carry the burden on his own shoulders - I would also like to thank his close friends and family who have helped him through this - my cousins Glen, Barrie and Ken (and their respective partners) who have kept in constant contact with emails and flowers - my Aunty Eva - Aunty Glad and Aunty Rhoda (who was visiting from Australia) who all rang me and sent me cards and flowers - my very old friend from way back (Jenny) who has also been there for me sending photos and emails (and her mum who I know has been asking after me) - my Personal Trainer at the gym who has sent me some truly touching emails - my friends in Birmingham and Bristol (Ellen and Jo who have been around me for the last 30 years) and I still cant get rid of them! To some of my neighbours (Peg and Derek) who have just been so sweet and thoughtful - knocking on the door to see how I am and bringing me lovely plants and choccie biscuits and cards - some of my work colleagues (even though we have all lost our jobs) who are still keeping in contact by mobile and text messages (Sue, Jackie, Kathy, Kelly and Yvonne) and again Jan (who I was in hospital with) we keep in regular contact just to make sure that our morale is kept at a high level. Even old friends of my mum and dad (Hylda and Bill) who have rung to give me support and words of encouragement. Stacey (Keith's daughter) who has phoned constantly to find out if I am ok and to be fair, my ex-husband Tony who has often phoned and given me words of comfort. If I have forgotten anyone at all I am truly sorry - and if I have - I also thank you so much for your support and helping me through this time in my life and I am so looking forward to March (which is when if all goes to plan my chemo will be over) and that is when I plan to have my Christmas Day Lunch with my family - so it is not December but that will not matter to any of us - just the fact that I have come through that awful tunnel and can now see the light again - even though I know in a few months time I will be going through radiotherapy - but you need something to look forward to and to push you forward and that is one of the things I want to achieve.

I would also like to thank all the ladies on Loose Women - I absolutely love the programme - my day revolves around it - I sit and have my roll and a bowl of soup and settle myself down - I have never known a programme that can have you in tears one minute (oh I so cried when Denise was going on about her hormone problem) and the next you are really laughing - my only complaint is that it is not on for long enough!

Also to thank Paul O'Grady and Alan Carr as I was bought those books as presents to make me sit and relax - and again what a tonic they both were - you realise that these men have gone through some dreadful times themselves and have ended up being a great success - fair play they certainly deserved it.

I know I am going to have to miss my grand-daughters first birthday - but I am sure she will understand and know that it has not been done deliberately and I will just have to ring her on that day.

It is now the 24th November and I am feeling very well - all ready to be hit again with the chemo tomorrow.

The only thing that is a bit of a "pain" at the moment is my head - it is very sore to touch and this morning it was really painful to brush or comb - and my hair is starting to come out quite a lot- not in clumps but in the comb and on to my clothes - having said that a lot of people get that every day when they brush their hair but I suppose it is more noticeable for me as it has never happened before - but I have just stuck a turban on my head today - not as if I am going anywhere or seeing anyone and if anyone comes to the door it looks as though you have just washed your hair!

Ellen stayed over on Tuesday and Wednesday and my father arrived Friday and left Sunday - but I must admit it was lovely to see them but I realise as well how tired I get - and again because I am looking and feeling so well I am continuing to do everything and I think by the end of the day you realise that you are really quite tired - but again a small price to pay.

The actual scar is healing really well and I can turn over in bed now and so can sleep on either side as well as my back - result!

Oh well I will be back again in about 5-6 days time just to let you know how it is going. It is now a week after the second lot of chemo - over 10 hours we were up the hospital waiting - we got there at 9.15 am and left at 7.45 - felt absolutely exhausted.

It seemed to take effect quicker this time - in fact on about the 3rd day I was feeling really tearful - Keith and I had a few words which is most unusual - but it seems as though my tolerance levels and patience levels are non existent at the moment - everything seems to be annoying me - especially the television - it seems as though the people who put these programmes out on the air think we are all just "brain dead" - I know I possibly am at this moment in time but not 100% brain dead.

I have felt very tearful - my hair is coming out in handfuls and my head is very painful and hair sore to brush (so I am going to buy a baby brush today) it even hurts my head to shower - very flu like and very spaced out - but I have totally given in to it - I do not want to make myself a hero but end up worse off - so I have just gone off to bed and slept whenever I have felt like it and it has obviously paid off because this morning I feel really well (even though I still have a bit of a flu type feeling in the head) so I am going to have a wander round Sainsburys - what an exciting morning to look forward to - but at least I am able to do it.

I have my next chemo on Tuesday 16th December, so I am hoping that I should have a reasonable Christmas - but at least we do not have too much planned - would rather not plan anything than plan something then have to cancel.

CHAPTER 9

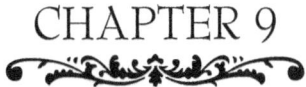

Well, I am still hanging on in there and at least after the next chemo session I will be half way through - then two in January and one in February and then that should be it before the radiotherapy - in fact we went and got some Travel Brochures last weekend - we are certainly planning on having a holiday as soon as this is all over - not only for me but for Keith as well - as I have said previously - this has been a very traumatic time for him also and he has taken the brunt of it when I have not felt too good

My daughter is still being as supportive - coming up whenever she can - telling me that I look young and pretty - which even though is probably not true it does make me feel better - in fact I suppose at the moment I have a Posh Becs hairstyle - and she has got all that money and wealth and she is still moaning about her short hair (what does she think the likes of us have to cope with) these celebrities really make me cross sometimes - they have so much and they just cannot see it - it is not until you have a health issue that you get your life into perspective and it is about time these wealthy people thought a little bit more about the good things they have. It is like me - yes I am having a real problem with the short hair at the moment - but unlike Posh - I have to get on with it - she could afford to go anywhere at anytime and get her hair sorted out - wake up and smell the coffee eh!!

It is now Tuesday 15th and it is my 3rd chemo session tomorrow - will just be glad when it is February and it is all over - but in all fairness I am doing quite well really - almost bald at the back now and very little hair on top - but at least I still have my fringe so that helps with the hat wearing.

My son came up with the family on Saturday - and it was time to wear the wig I thought - paid off - as no one realised that I was wearing one - as my fringe and the wig are exactly the same colour - and they all said how fantastic I looked and so well - so that puts a smile on your face.

I am watching all these programmes and everyone is saying that they are so excited about Christmas and they cant wait to see all the family and exchange presents - and I must admit I have had a few tears this last couple of weeks - seem to be far more weepy this time - the slightest thing sets me off and I just sob some times - but then once out the way I am fine again.

I did have a bit of a blow this morning though - as I had to see my doctor about another matter and I did ask her when after the chemotherapy and radiotherapy would I be given the "all clear" - and she told me that I would never be given the all clear and it would only take a small seed of cancer to hide itself and rear its ugly head in the future - as she said - it may not - but it can never be ruled out - and there was me thinking that once I had all the treatments that would give me a clear run - so had a few tears on that one when I got home - but went out and cleaned the car and did the washing and made a casserole and again I was fine after that.

I will be in contact again in a few weeks - after the 3rd session and I will let you know what sort of Christmas we had - I am sure it is going to be absolutely fantastic - in fact we will make sure it is.

Not too happy with the 3rd session - the nurse really hurt me - the first one doing the blood test and the oncologist really hurt - in fact bruised all my hand and an awful dark blue vein going up my arm - was that concerned I went to see the Pharmacist to ask his opinion - he said he did not think it was anything to worry about but just very bruised - it is now the 30th December and the arm still feels bruised although the bruises are no longer visible - hope I don't get her again - did not like her at all - and the fact that she just kept walking away and leaving me there - I know they are really rushed - too many patients for not enough staff but it does not instill much confidence in you when you are just left there. I did mention it to the oncologist I had on the 4th session and she said never leave anything like that - go straight back to Oncology - she said it sounded as though she caused a thrombosis!

After effects much about the same - although I do feel a lot more tired now - but having said that we did put up the small Christmas tree in the conservatory and the large one in the lounge - and we did get a visit from my son and daughter (and her parents) and my little grand-daughter - so that was lovely - and she appreciated the trees even if no one else did!

Not too good leading up to Christmas - but by Christmas Eve I was feeling a lot better and helped Keith prepare all the vegetables and Christmas morning I woke up as bright as a button - my daughter arrived about 8.30 that morning and Keith went for his mum about 11.30 (after having visited his own family) and we had a really enjoyable Christmas Day.

I am still feeling quite tired at the moment - but a week today is my 4th chemo session with only two more to go after that - and to be honest I cannot wait to get them out of the way - it is so unlike me to not be full of energy and be charging about - I am reading so many books these days it is unbelievable (thanks to Sue) - but - if that is what it takes then so be it - and I must say it is nice not to have to turn out on the cold frosty mornings to go work - I can get up whenever I want - go to bed whenever I want - and the resting certainly does help. I must admit the day times are ok, but it is at night, the brain just wont seem to switch off and your head is just buzzing constantly and I kept feeling when my eyes were closed that I was traveling through a vortex – I kept seeing vivid lime greens, yellows and purples – it was very pretty but quite frightening.

It is now Wednesday 14th January - and I am feeling really down and sorry for myself. Not sure if it is just the chemo or the fact that people are beginning to annoy me. We have had a personal problem within the family and it appears to me that no-one is really interested in any one else but themselves and it has really upset me - I don't want to do a "Jade" and publish to the world how I am feeling - but the chemo seemed to have hit me a bit harder this time - more emotional - and a couple of the days it has been a real struggle to get out of bed or do anything at all - and yet - there is my husband and I running ourselves ragged and everyone else just sitting back and letting us - what is the matter with people today?

Sorry - did say I was on a bit of a downer - did not help yesterday either when I had a delivery - and of course not thinking as I am so used to being in the house without a wig or a hat I just automatically answered the door - this poor delivery man looked horrified - I think he felt he was on a set for Lord of the Rings - so I took my parcel - thanked him - closed the door - and burst into tears and sobbed for quite a while - thinking - what an absolute freak you look - no hair -

no boobs - nothing - but fortunately that has passed today and I have been out and done some shopping and made myself feel better and am really looking forward to spending a few days with my daughter - as she always tells me I look lovely.

I have got my dad coming in a few weeks as he seems quite upset that he has not seen me for a while - but I did warn him last night that I am not the prettiest of sights and I don't want him to get upset when he sees me - I don't think people realise how low your ego goes - and you do try to put on a false image but I don't want to do that anymore - I am fed up with people thinking that I am fit and well - and I am not.

It is now Monday 26th January (and it is my 5th chemo tomorrow) and I have just had a lovely weekend. My dad came on the Friday and on the Saturday we went down to my grand-daughters (Elissa's) birthday - so I made it - I did not think I would - she is such a little cutie and we had a lovely time - only stayed a few hours as I start to get a bit weary after that and then on the Sunday we went to a lovely Restaurant for lunch and then my dad headed back to Devon as it would then give us the evening and the next day for me to relax before my next session.

I think my dad was quite surprised - as when he arrived I was not wearing a hat or a wig - I thought I would let him see the real me as I am at the moment - but when I got made up and dressed and put the wig on the next day to go to the birthday party, I don't think he could believe it was the same person - what a transformation - and in fact everyone said how well I looked - so that made me feel 100% better.

I am just counting down the days now - got quite tearful this morning as I am beginning to realise that we are now nearing the end of the chemo and hopefully by April the radiotherapy will also be over - I can then start planning my life again - but every morning I wake up I am so grateful.

It is now Thursday 12th February and two weeks after my 5th chemo - and I must say it has hit me a bit harder this time - in fact on Wednesday 4th because I had the mouth ulcers in my mouth and throat for over a week my daughter begged me to ring the Chemo Help Line - which I did - they told me to go straight to Hospital (this was 8.00 at night) - when I got there they told me that if I had anything like that again to ring the Helpline immediately as it could be a sign of infection and in fact you could be dead within two hours - well my blood pressure was 213/119 - why were they so surprised - I had just had a terrible shock - so out came the ECG machine - they took my bloods to check for my liver and kidney and blood count - but fortunately by 11.00 pm I was allowed to go home - I have never felt so relieved.

Once again the mother in law went back into Hospital on Monday (she has been in and out of Hospital since December) - so Tuesday I was round changing the bed and getting her washing - then on Wednesday went round and tidied up and vacuumed - Wednesday afternoon went into Hospital to visit - and by this morning (Thursday) I am absolutely shattered - I feel so tired - so I am going to have a restful day today - and if anything else needs doing round her place someone else will just have to do it from now on I cannot afford to end up in Hospital myself at this late stage. I thought maybe her own daughter may have helped out – but it seemed as though there was no chance of that – makes me really cross – I would give anything to be able to go and visit my mum – why can people see they do not know what they have until it is gone!

Anyway - at least things are still going well and most of the time I do feel quite fit but you know that you cannot fight it and it is not worth it - so when the body tells you to rest - that is what you do.

I had my last chemo this Tuesday 17th - what a relief - although it was the worst one I had experienced to date - I had Margaret as my chemo nurse and she had problems getting the canular in twice - so then had to pass me over to another nurse who managed to succeed - but I did start to feel really sick as the needles were stinging and it was really uncomfortable - but once again my daughter was there to support me - and I really don't know what I would have done without her throughout this ordeal - she is the only one as well that they have allowed to sit in with me - and considering she hates needles etc this has been an extremely hard time for her as well. They dont normally like people being with you as the rooms are quite crowded with the machinery, the patients and the oncologists and also for infection reasons – so I was really grateful for the staff who allowed her to sit with me.

It is now Thursday 19th - and I really did not have a very good day yesterday - seemed all right in the morning but by the afternoon I began to feel really sick - and I was - so I decided to come back to bed for the afternoon but I felt very nauseas and continued to keep being sick - I took my temperature and everything seemed to be all right - as Margaret gave me a good telling off that I had not rung the Helpline on previous occasions and she told me how extremely dangerous it was if you had the symptoms on your Helpline List if you did not contact them - and that is exactly what they were they for.

Poor Keith - was torn between me and his mum - as she is still in hospital awaiting now to undergo a bladder operation - and he rang me and asked if I would like him to come straight home - I told him that I was perfectly OK as long as I was laying still and I thought it best he go and visit his mum – as she is nearly 90.

He arrived home a bit later - and for once had to get his own meal - I had prepared half of it but when I went to complete it the nausea took over! But he came and sat with me on the bed for a while - I then had another bout of sickness and after that I did not feel too bad - I did sleep in the spare room as I felt I was not going to have a good night - which I didn't - I just closed my eyes and just wanted to go to sleep but it would not come and my stomach was creaking and groaning, but when I woke up this morning I felt OK - stomach felt a little sore but the headache and the nausea had passed - but I decided to take it easy and stayed in bed until mid-day - the sun is now shining and it is a beautiful day - but I have just watched the news (and I am extremely emotional with the chemo - in fact I still cry during some adverts!) and of course the news of Jade came on and the preparation for her wedding this weekend - that poor girl - I must admit I have never really taken to her but I would certainly not wish what she has on anyone and I hope that she manages to stay well enough to walk down the aisle and I am sure will make everyone proud of her.

I do say that unless you have undergone the chemotherapy (and I have now been told I have to have 13 sessions of radiotherapy starting on the 17th March) you cannot describe to anyone the feelings that you get with it - once the chemicals are administered - the side effects - the horrendous part when you can see more hair on the side than you have on your head and just not being able to feel as though you are in control of anything - and so again my heart goes out to the girl - as although I am suffering in my own way I don't think I am going through anywhere near what she is going through at this point in time. We all know now that unfortunately she did not make it – her poor children.

CHAPTER 10

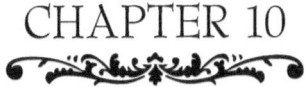

My daughter has now got a new man in her life and he sounds absolutely wonderful and I have seen such a change in her since she has been seeing him - it has been just over a month now and it could not have come at a better time for me - and of course for her - as she now has someone that she can turn to when things get worrying for her over me - and just for someone to love and take care of her as she is so special and she deserves the very best and I wish her and Adam all the very best for the future - and I hope there is a future - but should things go wrong for any reason - and I do not think that they should - I will remove this part from the book before it is published! If not - watch this space and I will let you know how and when things progress - this has also given me such a wonderful feeling and Keith and I are so ecstatically happy for her. The news is they are getting married on 17th July 2010.

I go for my pre-radiotherapy on Thursday 12th March which is when they mark up the body to zap you - but I am not as fearful of this as I was before I started the chemo - I must admit these six sessions have really gone quite quickly and even though I have had my rough days and my very tearful days it was not nearly as bad as I thought it was going to be.

It is now Friday 27th February and this is the first day since my last chemo on Tuesday 17th that I can say I actually have started to feel human again.

I was quite bad on the Tuesday - very sick and again on the Wednesday and Thursday and Friday although I was not being sick I felt very nauseas. By the Saturday my body felt as though it had gone into complete shut down and I felt absolutely lousy and very tearful - and I must admit for the first time I can say I actually felt frightened - I did not think I was going to pull out of this one. On the Saturday morning at about 2.00 am I was beginning to think I was going to have to be taken to the Hospital - I felt so ill. I could not sleep - my brain would not seem to shut off and although I was so tired I could not sleep - or was it I did not want to - I really was scared that if I went into a deep sleep I would not wake up again. On the Sunday at 10.30 I decided to ring the Helpline as I really thought I was on my way out - but they asked me to see how I felt by 1.00 - by that time I started to feel a bit better - I don't know whether it was the fear of having to be admitted to hospital and it was purely psychological. So I did not go down - by about 4.30 it hit me again but this time it was a strange feeling and I just felt as though I wanted to close my eyes and just shut everything out - I managed to cook a Sunday roast - which I could not manage to eat but needless to say Keith had no problem - it seemed as though every time I ate something solid it just seemed to go straight through me. At 8.00 I decided to go back to bed.

On the Monday I woke up feeling a little bit brighter - my body had seemed to return to me and from that day on it just seems to have started to feel more human like.

My daughter came up yesterday (Thursday) and again we had a lovely chatty day - she filed and painted my nails for me - we went and did a bit of shopping and she left about 3.30 and I just felt on such a high - she had bought me some lovely lead-crystal candle holders (so we had to go out and buy some candles) and as she left I just watched the flame - so peaceful and calm and I felt really well.

So as I said, it is now Friday morning - the sun is shining - my hair is already starting to grow back - not only on my head but also my legs and arms, but I have never been so grateful to see hair growing and I can now say that the chemotherapy is over and hopefully my body will now return back to me fully charged - I realise now that I am still over-weight so I have started doing some exercises - I am going to continue to eat healthily - fortunately the chemo completely put me off alcohol this time so that has helped - but I must admit I will probably have a glass of wine this weekend as I want to stop drinking again completely when I have the radiotherapy - and with a bit of luck during that five weeks I can start to lose some of this unwanted weight - I think it has always been there but owing to the fact that I had such big boobs it was not always possible to see the bulge that lay beneath - so I have been given another chance and I want to make sure I make the most of it.

It is now Monday 9th March and I am just relaxing after having my dad here for the weekend - I am still getting quite tired but I am feeling really well at the moment and I am hoping that it will stay that way.

I will let you know how the radiotherapy goes and give you an update on the hair growth and hopefully the weight loss!

Well it is now a week since the radiotherapy finished and I am feeling really well. Had a few ups and downs with the radiotherapy and the Arimidex - had a terrible nose bleed that we could not stop but I did not feel as tired and washed out as they said I would - my skin is also quite burnt and itchy but they said that would improve about ten days after the treatment. My hair is now growing back quite well - do not feel confident enough to go out yet without a wig but at least it is growing back.

I had to go and see the Consultant this week as the Arimidex was causing me to have rheumatism type side effects which were really painful and keeping me awake at night. I must admit that I was quite disappointed in the attitude of the Consultant from start to finish – he seemed very abrupt and not very caring. The very first appointment we had with him he seemed very distant – did not shake our hands when he came in and when finished with us he just walked out of the room – we all sat there wondering if he was coming back! He was not very sympathetic when I told him about the side effects and he just said "well what do you want me to do about it" – what! He is the Consultant – and then he said "well you have to take something" – well I appreciate that – then he said that the side effects really had to be unbearable before they liked to change the tablets – I had undergone a Sentinel Lymph Gland operation – a double mastectomy – six sessions of chemotherapy and thirteen sessions of radiotherapy – I think my pain threshold was quite high! So he agreed to put me on the Tamoxifen – but then he said come and see me at your next session – I told him my sessions were now finished and he said "well when is your follow up appointment" – I told him I did not know as the Receptionist did not seem to have a record of it and he said "well that is not my fault". I felt so intimidated – I am not a patient who makes a fuss and keeps moaning and I just felt as though he was so insincere and uncaring. When I got out of the hospital I just burst into tears.

I now have to return on the 9th June for my review and I think it is then that I am given the "news" - so I will return once that session is over!!

It is now 15th June 2009 and this will be the final paragraph of my book - I was given the ALL CLEAR by the Consultant and I do not have to go back for another year.

You can imagine the elation - my daughter and Keith came with me and when we walked out of the Hospital we just had a group hug and a few tears - we then got home and opened up the champagne and a few more tears - it is a hard feeling to describe - it is almost like being reborn - it has just lifted that black cloud from above me and I feel as though I can live again.

I have lots to do within the next year - my daughter is getting married and I plan to lose about two stone for that day - I am joining Weight Watchers today - I have taken out a mini membership at the gym and I am going jogging three times a week (all ok at the moment until I get a job hopefully). I am determined to see this through - and to be given another chance in life just gives you that extra incentive that you needed.

This has been the worst journey of my life and I certainly would not like to have to do it again - but if anyone is reading this book - is ever told that they have cancer - please do not give up - and when you are offered the treatments - take them - they are not very nice but if they save your life it is worth it - I almost backed out from having them - especially the chemotherapy - but to be honest it is like having a baby - yes it is painful whilst in labour but once the baby is born the pain is forgotten - it is like the chemotherapy - not very nice when you are going through it - but once it is over it is over.

I am just so thankful to be given a second chance and once again I would like to thank each and everyone of you who stood by me and supported me through my awful ordeal - I will never forget any of you - and you certainly find out who your true friends are.

Just to keep you up to date – the hair is growing quite nicely now – still quite short but come back really thick, dark and a little wavey – and yes I did go out shopping yesterday without the wig! Everyone is saying how fantastic I look.

I have been at Weightwatchers now for two weeks and have lost five pounds in weight – that is an incentive to keep going. I am jogging every morning now and I intend to go swimming twice a week – I will get into the nice outfit for my daughter's wedding!

We went to Bulgaria for a week on the 24th August and we now have a holiday booked for the 10th September to Greece.

My little grandson Jayden was born just as we got back from holiday and I am so proud to be a grandmother again and to have been able to hold him when he was just a few days old.

We have celebrated our first wedding anniversary and what a year it has been – I cannot believe that the time has passed so quickly.

I had to see the Surgeon and the scar and my liver was examined and everything is fine – I don't have to go back now for another six months. I have been on the Tamoxifen now for a few months and the only side effects seem to be the hot flushes! Not too bad throughout the day but at night! I am probably only getting about three to four hours sleep – it is that bad it wakes me up – my hair, face and neck are absolutely soaked – it only lasts about ten minutes but it disturbs your sleep – but if that is my only problem then I am prepared to live with it. I am pleased I did no go with the reconstruction.

I am happy with the way I look and the way I feel – and when you are out in company – either with the prosthesis or not – no-one ever knows that you are any different to any other woman. My only fear now is not for myself but for my daughter– as she is obviously high-risk but they have told her that they will not screen her until she is 30 – so I have everything crossed that she will forever be clear!

On my return home there was a delivery of flowers – a beautiful bouquet of white carnations and white roses from Nicki and Adam – what an absolutely perfect end to my journey!

www.ingramcontent.com/pod-product-compliance
Lightning Source LLC
Chambersburg PA
CBHW021250280526
45784CB00005B/2316